CW00657316

The Complete Mediterranean Diet Cookbook For Beginners

A Quick Guide To Complete Mediterranean Diet Guide With Delicious Recipes And A Meal Plan To Help You Get Started

By

Grace Morelli

Copyright 2021 - All rights reserved.

The content contained within this book may not be reproduced, duplicated or transmitted without direct written permission from the author or the publisher.

Under no circumstances will any blame or legal responsibility be held against the publisher, or author, for any damages, reparation, or monetary loss due to the information contained within this book. Either directly or indirectly.

Legal Notice:

This book is copyright protected. This book is only for personal use. You cannot amend, distribute, sell, use, quote or paraphrase any part, or the content within this book, without the consent of the author or publisher.

Disclaimer Notice:

Please note the information contained within this document is for educational and entertainment purposes only. All effort has been executed to present accurate, up to date, and reliable, complete information. No warranties of any kind are declared or implied. Readers acknowledge that the author is not engaging in the rendering of legal, financial, medical or professional advice. The content within this book has been derived from various sources. Please consult a licensed professional before attempting any techniques outlined in this book.

By reading this document, the reader agrees that under no circumstances is the author responsible for any losses, direct or indirect, which are incurred as a result of the use of information contained within this document, including, but not limited to, errors, omissions, or inaccuracies.

Table Of Contents

Introduction

Thank you very much for purchasing this book. After the "Study of the seven countries" by Ancel Keys, conducted since the 1950s, research on the Mediterranean diet has multiplied, leading to a detailed understanding of the effect of the intake of certain foods on health. If the food pyramid is the model with which to describe the Mediterranean diet, today there is no single version and, in some cases, the differences are related to the age of those who must use it. The common aspect of these diets is that they all aim to introduce healthy and nutritious foods into one's diet. Thanks to the Mediterranean diet it is possible to lose weight and drastically reduce the risk of cardiovascular disease. I hope my recipes can help you improve your lifestyle.

Enjoy your meal.

Mediterranean Smoothies Recipes

Sweet Smoothie

(Prep time: 10 minutes | Blend time: 2 minutes |Servings: 1)

Nutrition: 103 Cal | 8.3 g Fat |11.2 g Carbs | 6 g Protein

Ingredients

- Fresh pineapple: 1 cup

- 1 banana

- Coconut water: half cup

- 1 mango: sliced

Instructions

- Add all ingredients to the blender. Pulse on high until smooth and creamy.

- Serve right away.

Coconut Blueberry Smoothie

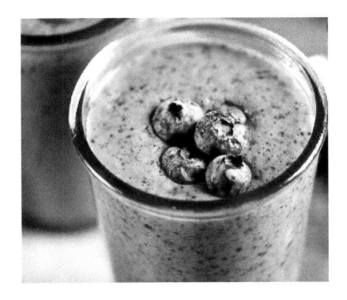

(Prep time: 10 minutes | Blend time: 2 minutes |Servings: 1)

Nutrition: 103 Cal | 8 g Fat |21 g Carbs |16 g Protein

Ingredients

- Macadamia nut milk: 1 cup

- Vanilla protein powder: 1 scoop

- 2 chunks of frozen coconut

- Frozen blueberries: 1 cup

Instructions

- Add all ingredients to the blender. Pulse on high until smooth and creamy.

- Serve right away

Coffee Smoothie

(Prep time: 10 minutes | Blend time: 2 minutes |Servings: 1)

Nutrition: 161 Cal | 7 g Fat |33 g Carbs |3 g Protein

Ingredients

- Fat-free milk: ¼ cup

- Coffee powder, instant espresso: 1 tsp.

- Honey: 1 tbsp.

- Ice cubes: half cup

- Hot water: 1 tbsp.

- 1 frozen banana

Instructions

- Add all ingredients to the blender. Pulse on high until smooth and creamy.

- Serve right away.

Mediterranean Breakfast Recipes

Loaded Mediterranean Omelette

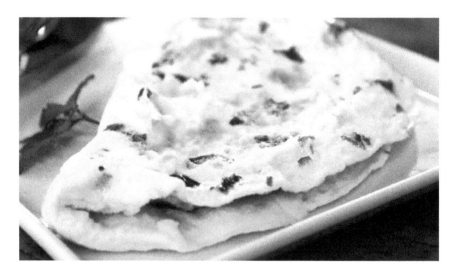

(Prep time:5 minutes | Cook time: 10 minutes |Servings: 2)

Nutrition: 109 Cal | 12 g Fat |23 g Carbs |16.9 g Protein

Ingredients

- Milk: 2 tbsp.

- Salt & black pepper, to taste

- Baking powder: ¼ tsp.

- 4 eggs

- Spanish paprika: half tsp.

- Tzatziki sauce, as required

- Ground allspice: ¼ tsp.

- Olive oil: 1 ½ tsp

Toppings

- Artichoke hearts (marinated): ¼-⅓ cup, drained & quartered

- Cherry tomatoes: half cup, halved

- Fresh mint: 2 tbsp., chopped

- Sliced Kalamata olives: 2 tbsp.

- Fresh parsley: 2 tbsp., chopped

Instructions

- In a bowl, whisk eggs with baking powder, salt, spices, milk and pepper.

- In a skillet, add oil and pour the egg mixture (some of it) when it gets hot.

- Immediately stir the eggs and pour more, repeat the mixture until eggs are cooked.

- Turn off the heat and add your preferred toppings in the lower part; fold the omelet around the toppings.

- Cut in half and serve with fresh herbs on top and with tzatziki sauce.

Easy, Fluffy Lemon Pancakes

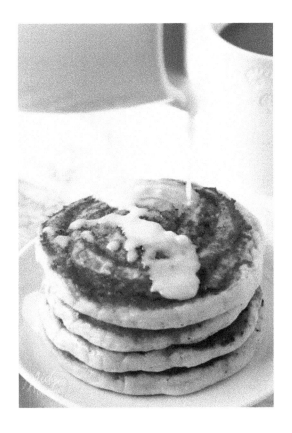

(Prep time: 10 minutes | Cook time: 20 minutes |Servings: 4)

Nutrition: 344 Cal | 15.9 g Fat |32.1 g Carbs |17.1 g Protein

Ingredients

- Baking powder: 1 tsp.

- 4 eggs

- Ricotta cheese: 1 cup

- 2% milk: half cup

- Granulated sugar: 1 tbsp.

- 1 lemon

- All-purpose flour: 1 cup

- Kosher salt: 1/4 tsp.

Instructions

- In different bowls, separate whites and yolks.

- In the egg yolk, add lemon zest and lemon juice.

- Add milk and ricotta cheese whisk well.

- Add the rest of the ingredients mix until just combined.

- With a stand mixer, whisk the egg whites for 2-3 minutes until stiff peaks form.

- Fold the egg whites into the yolk mixture.

- In a skillet, add enough butter to coat the pan and add ¼ cup of batter.

- Cook for 2-3 minutes on each side and serve with maple syrup.

Grain Bowl with Sautéed Spinach

(Prep time: 5 minutes | Cook time: 5 minutes |Servings: 2)

Nutrition: 458 Cal | 21 g Fat |52 g Carbs |14 g Protein

Ingredients

- Spinach: 4 cups, roughly chopped

- Cooked grains: 2 cups

- 1 minced garlic clove

- 2 eggs

- Olive oil: 1 tbsp.

- Kosher salt: 1/4 tsp.

- Half avocado, diced

- Pepper: 1/4 tsp.

- 1 tomato, cut into small pieces

Instructions

- In bowls, add warmed grains.

- In a skillet, add oil, garlic and cook for 1 minute.

- Add spinach and season with salt and pepper, cook for 1-2 minutes.

- Put on top of grains with avocado and tomato.

- Cook egg to your desired doneness. Serve the bowls with eggs on top.

Cauliflower Fritters With Hummus

(Prep time: 10 minutes | Cook time: 50 minutes |Servings: 4)

Nutrition: 251 Cal | 20 g Fat |24 g Carbs |17 g Protein

Ingredients

- Cauliflower: 2 cups, broken into smaller pieces

- 1 can of (15 oz.) Chickpeas

- Chopped Onion: 1 cup

- Black Pepper, to taste

- Minced garlic: 2 tbsp.

- Olive Oil: 2 1/2 tbsp.

- Salt: half tsp.

Instructions

- Let the oven preheat to 400 F.

- Dry the chickpeas (half of the can) well, put them in a large bowl, and toss with olive oil (1 tbsp.).

- Spread on a baking tray, season with salt and black pepper. Bake for 20-35 minutes until crispy. Take chickpeas out on a plate

- Place roasted chickpeas in a food processor, and pulse until crumbly and broken down. Do not make it into powder.

- In a skillet, add the oil and sauté garlic, onion for 2 minutes.

- Add cauliflower and cook for 2 minutes more until it is golden.

- Cover the pan and turn the heat low; cook for 3 to 5 minutes, until fork-tender.

- Put this cauliflower in the food processor, add the rest of the chickpeas and blend until smooth and becomes one.

- Take out in a bowl and half cup of the crumbly chickpeas. Mix well.

- Make into patties and cook these patties in a pan for 2 to 3 minutes on each side.

- Serve with hummus and enjoy.

Baked Eggs in Avocado

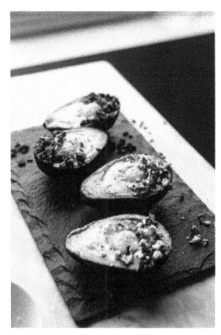 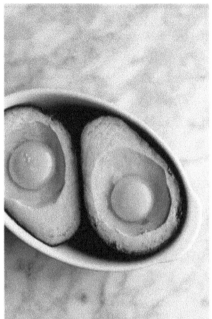

(Prep time: 10 minutes | Cook time: 15 minutes | Servings: 2)

Nutrition: 251 Cal | 20 g Fat | 24 g Carbs | 17 g Protein

Ingredients

- Chopped fresh chives: 2 tsp.

- 2 eggs

- 1 avocado, halved and emptied

- Dried parsley, to taste

- Cooked bacon: 2 slices, crumbled

- Salt & black pepper, to taste

Instructions

- Let the oven preheat to 425 F.

- In a bowl, add eggs, do no break the yolks.

- In a baking dish, arrange avocado halves, add one yolk in each half, and pour enough white to fill the shell.

- Season with salt, chives, parsley and pepper.

- Put the baking dish in the oven and cook for 15 minutes, serve with bacon on top.

- Gently place the baking dish in the preheated oven and bake until eggs are cooked about 15 minutes. Sprinkle bacon over avocado.

Mediterranean Poultry Recipes

Greek-Style Stuffed Peppers

(Prep time: 30 minutes| Cook time: 4-5 ½ hours|Servings: 8)

Nutrition: 313 Cal | 16 g Fat |26 g Carbs |17 g Protein

Ingredients

- Pack of (10 oz.) spinach, dry

- olive oil: 2 tbsp.

- 1 can of (28 oz.) crushed tomatoes, divided

- 1 red onion, diced

- 2 minced garlic cloves

- 2 sweet oranges, red, green & yellow peppers

- Salt: half tsp.

- 1 fennel bulb, diced

- 1 pound of ground chicken

- Cooked barley: 1 cup

- Pepper: half tsp.

- Greek olives: half cup, chopped

- Crumbled feta cheese: 1 cup

- Dried oregano: 1 to 1/2 tsp.

- Red pepper flakes: half tsp.

Instructions

- In a pan, sauté onion, fennel in hot oil over medium flame, cook for 6 to 8 minutes.

- Add garlic, spinach cook for 1 minute. Turn off the heat and let it cool.

- Cut the tops off of peppers, and take out the middle part.

- In the slow cooker (6-7 qt.), add crushed tomatoes (1 cup).

- In a bowl, add chicken, seasonings, olives, barley, fennel mixture and feta cheese (1 cup). Mix and spoon into peppers.

- Place the peppers in the slow cooker, and put the tops on.

- Cook for 4 to 5 ½ hours till peppers are tender.

- Serve with feta on top.

Turkey & Black Bean Taco Casserole

(Prep time: 10 minutes| Cook time: 30 minutes|Servings: 6)

Nutrition: 298 Cal | 10 g Fat |24 g Carbs |29 g Protein

Ingredients

- Green onions: 1 cup, chopped

- Riced cauliflower: 2 cups

- Ground turkey breast: 1 pound

- Ground cumin: 1 tsp.

- Fresh cilantro: 2 tbsp., chopped

- Canola oil: 1 tbsp.

- Kosher salt: half tsp.

- Chili powder: 1 tsp.

- Garlic powder: 1 tsp.

- 1 can of (15 oz.) black beans, rinsed

- Smoked paprika: half tsp.

- Cherry tomatoes: 1 cup, chopped

- Tomato sauce: 1 cup

- Corn kernels: 1 cup

- Colby jack cheese: 1 cup, grated

- Lime juice: 1 tsp.

Instructions

- Let the oven preheat to 425 F.

- In a skillet, add oil on medium flame.

- Add green onions (half cup) and turkey, cook for four minutes.

- Add riced cauliflower, smoked paprika, cumin, chili powder and garlic. Cook for 3 to 4 minutes.

- Add salt and tomato sauce, cook for 1 to 2 minutes.

- In a casserole dish (2 qt.), add cooked turkey mixture, layer corn, black beans and cheese on top.

- Bake for 15 minutes until cheese is bubbly.

- In a bowl, add the rest of the ingredients, mix and pour over casserole. Serve right away.

Crispy Spatchcock Chicken

(Prep time: 15 minutes| Cook time: 50 minutes|Servings: 6)

Nutrition: 404 Cal | 7.5 g Fat |6.9 g Carbs |33.3 g Protein

Ingredients

- Whole chicken: 4 lb.

- Sweet paprika: half tsp.

- Salt, to taste

- Garlic powder: 1 ½ tsp.

- Olive oil, as needed

- Black pepper: half tsp.

- Allspice: 1 ½ tsp.

- Ground nutmeg: ¼ tsp.

Instructions

- Butterfly the chicken, or ask your butcher to do it for you.

- Season the chicken with salt on both sides. Keep in the fridge for few hours.

- Before cooking, let it rest and come to room temperature.

- Let the oven preheat to 425 F.

- In a bowl, mix all spices and coat the chicken well. Season underneath the skin too.

- In a skillet, add enough oil to coat the pan and brown the chicken for 5-8 minutes on each side.

- Place the skillet in the oven, bake for 20 minutes.

- After 20 minutes, rotate the skillet and cook for 30-45 minutes, until the chicken is completely cooked until the internal temperature of the meat reaches 165 F.

- Serve with roasted vegetables.

Turkey Bowl With Lemony Vinaigrette

(Prep time: 25 minutes| Cook time: 0 minutes|Servings: 4)

Nutrition: 312 Cal | 7.6 g Fat |19 g Carbs |23 g Protein

Ingredients

Lemony Vinaigrette

- Each salt & black pepper: ¼ tsp.

- Lemon juice: 3 tbsp.

- Red pepper flakes, a pinch

- Dried oregano: 1 tsp.

- Olive oil: ⅓ cup

- 2 minced garlic clove

Nourish Bowl

- English cucumber: 2 cups, half-moons

- Grape tomatoes: 2 cups, halved

- Canned chickpeas: 1 cup, rinsed

- Cubed turkey: 2 cups, cooked

- Yellow pepper: 2 cups, chopped

- Kalamata olives: 4 tbsp., sliced

- Red onion: ¼ cup, diced

- Cooked barley: 2 cups,

- Crumbled feta cheese: ⅓ cup

Instructions

- In a bowl, add all ingredient of Vinaigrette, whisk well and set it aside.

- In four bowls, divide the rest of the ingredients. Pour over vinaigretter and serve.

Greek Sun-Dried Tomato Chicken & Farro

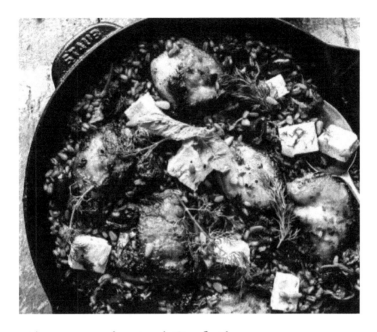

(Prep time: 15 minutes| Cook time: 40 minutes|Servings: 6)

Nutrition: 324 Cal | 9.2 g Fat |20 g Carbs |22 g Protein

Ingredients

- Chicken breasts: 1 pound, boneless & skinless

- Olive oil: 1/4 cup

- Extra virgin olive oil: 2 tbsp.

- Fresh oregano: 1 tbsp., chopped

- Balsamic vinegar: 2 tbsp.

- Fresh dill: 1 tbsp., chopped

- Paprika: 1 tbsp.

- 2 minced garlic cloves

- Salt & black pepper, to taste

- Farro: 1 cup, uncooked

- Fresh dill: 1 tbsp.

- Kalamata olives: 1/3 cup, pitted

- Chicken broth: 2 1/2 cups

- Baby spinach: 2 cups

- 1 lemon's juice

- Sun-dried tomatoes: half cup, oil-packed

- Feta cheese: 1 cup, cubed

Instructions

- Let the oven preheat to 400 F.

- In a bowl, add chicken, all spices and herbs with 2 tbsp. of oil. Coat the chicken well.

- In a pan, add oil (2 tbsp.) on medium flame. Sear the chicken for 3 to 5 minutes on each side. Take the chicken out on a plate.

- In the same pan, add farro. Cook for 2 to 3 minutes, add the rest of the ingredients, mix and let it come to a boil.

- Add the chicken back in and put it in the oven.

- Bake for 20 minutes.

- Serve right away.

Mediterranean Appetizers & Sides Recipes

Greek Cauliflower Rice

(Prep time: 10 minutes | Cook time: 0 minutes |Servings: 8)

Nutrition: 109 Cal | 9 g Fat |6 g Carbs | 3g Protein

Ingredients

- English cucumber: half cup, chopped

- 1 Cauliflower, small head, broken into florets

- Diced red onion: half cup

- Minced garlic: 1 tbsp.

- Olive oil: 2 tbsp.

- Halved grape tomatoes: 1 cup

- Chopped walnuts: ¼ cup

- Crumbled feta cheese: half cup

- Halved Kalamata olives: half cup

- Fresh parsley: ¼ cup, chopped

- Black pepper: ¼ tsp.

- 1 lemon's juice & zest

- Fine sea salt: ¼ tsp.

Instructions

- In the instant pot, add water (1 cup), place the trivet in the pot, place cauliflower in it.

- Shut the lid, and close the valve (pressure-release). Set for 0 minutes (it mean it does not require much time but build pressure) & on high.

- After that, quick-release pressure. Take cauliflower out in a bowl.

- In the instant pot, drain any liquid, select sauté. Add oil and sauté garlic for four minutes. Cancel the sauté. Add cauliflower to the pot and mash with a masher into rice-like consistency.

- Take cauliflower out in a bowl, add the rest of the ingredients and toss well.

- Season with salt and black pepper.

Hummus Wraps

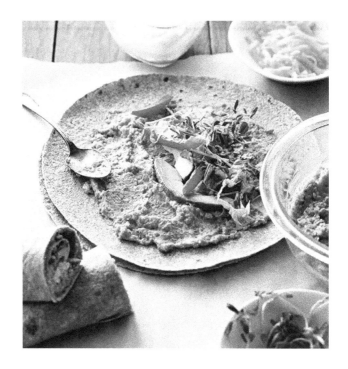

(Prep time: 10 minutes | Cook time: 0 minutes |Servings: 1)

Nutrition: 142 Cal | 6 g Fat |17 g Carbs | 6 g Protein

Ingredients

- Yellow onions: 1/4 cup, chopped

- 1 Whole grain tortilla, medium

- Dino kale: 1 cup

- Hummus: 1/4 cup

- Chopped tomatoes: 1/4 cup

- Half avocado

Instructions

- Place tortilla on a surface, and spread hummus all over.

- Add the rest of the ingredients on top.

- Fold into a burrito. Cut in half and serve.

Tuna Protein Box

(Prep time: 10 minutes | Cook time: 0 minutes |Servings: 2)

Nutrition: 414 Cal | 25 g Fat |20 g Carbs | 27 g Protein

Ingredients

* 4 hard-boiled eggs

* Grapes: 1 cup

* 4 carrots, chopped

* Cheese cubed: 8 oz.

* Celery: 2-3 ribs, chopped

* Blueberries: 1 cup

Tuna Salad

* Celery finely chopped: 2 tbsp.

* 1 Can of (5 oz.) Tuna, drained

* Salt & pepper, to taste

* Mayonnaise: 2 tbsp.

Instructions

- In a bowl, add all ingredients of tuna salad and mix.

- Take bento boxes, divide the salad in between them along with other ingredients and serve.

Greek Tuna Salad Bites

(Prep time: 10 minutes | Cook time: 0 minutes |Servings: 1)

Nutrition: 214 Cal | 13 g Fat |9.3 g Carbs | 21 g Protein

Ingredients

- Tuna: 6 oz., drained & flaked

- Red bell pepper: half cup (diced)

- Fresh parsley: 2 tbsp.

- 2 cucumbers, sliced

- Red onion: ¼ cup

- Half lemon

- Black olives: ¼ cup, chopped

- Minced garlic: 2 tbsp.

- Salt & black pepper, to taste

- Olive oil: 2 tbsp.

Instructions

- In a large bowl, add all ingredients, toss well and serve.

Mediterranean Fish & Seafood Recipes

Roasted Herb Salmon

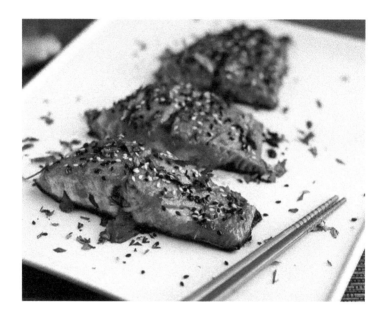

(Prep time: 10 minutes | Cook time: 10 minutes |Servings: 4)

Nutrition: 322 Cal | 20 g Fat | 6 g Carbs | 30 g Protein

Ingredients

- 4 salmon fillets

- Lemon juice: 2 tbsp.

- Chopped fresh thyme: 1 tbsp.

- Dijon mustard: 2 tbsp.

- 1 yellow onion, sliced thin

- Chopped fresh rosemary: 1 tbsp.

- Salt: half tsp.

- Dried oregano: 1 tsp.

- Black pepper: half tsp.

- 2 tomatoes, sliced thin

Instructions

- Make cuts on each fish fillet.

- In a bowl, add all spices and herbs. Mix well and coat the fish in it.

- Keep in the fridge for 15 minutes, covered with plastic wrap.

- Let the oven preheat to 450 F.

- Oil spray a baking pan and place vegetable slices on the bottom.

- Place fish on top. Bake for 10-15 minutes.

- Serve right away.

Greek Fish Bake

(Prep time: 10 minutes | Cook time: 20 minutes |Servings: 4)

Nutrition: 246 Cal | 12 g Fat | 6 g Carbs | 29 g Protein

Ingredients

- 4 cod fillets

- Pitted Greek olives: 1/4 cup, sliced

- 2 tablespoons olive oil: 2 tbsp.

- Salt: ¼ tsp.

- Crumbled feta cheese: 1/4 cup

- 1 green pepper, sliced into thin strips

- Pepper: 1/8 tsp.

- Half red onion, sliced thin

- 1 can of (8 oz.) tomato sauce

Instructions

- Let the oven preheat to 400 F.

- Oil spray a 13 by 9 baking tray, place fish inside and brush with olive oil.

- Season with salt and pepper. Add olives, onion and peppers on top.

- Add tomato sauce on top, with cheese.

- Bake for 15 to 20 minutes.

- Serve right away.

Spanish Garlic Shrimp

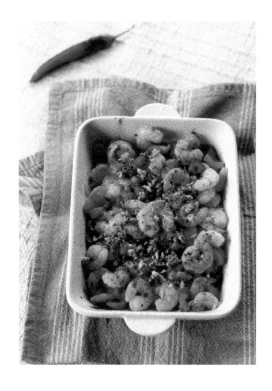

(Prep time: 10 minutes | Cook time: 20 minutes | Servings: 4)

Nutrition: 250 Cal | 17 g Fat | 3.4 g Carbs | 15.8 g Protein

Ingredients

- Olive oil: 1/3 cup

- Large shrimp: 1 pound, peeled & deveined

- 4 minced garlic cloves

- Chili flakes: ¼ tsp.

- Sweet Spanish paprika: 1 tsp.

- Lemon juice: 1 ½ tbsp.

- Kosher salt: ¼ tsp.

- Dry sherry: 2 tbsp.

- Pepper, to taste

- Chopped parsley: 2 tbsp.

Instructions

- In a pan, add oil and saute garlic with chili flakes on medium flame.

- Do not burn or brown the garlic. Add shrimp, season with salt, paprika and pepper.

- Cook for two minutes. Add lemon juice, sherry, cook for 2 to 3 minutes.

- Add parsley on top and serve.

Walnut-Rosemary Crusted Salmon

(Prep time: 10 minutes | Cook time: 10 minutes |Servings: 4)

Nutrition: 222 Cal | 12 g Fat | 4 g Carbs | 24 g Protein

Ingredients

- Dijon mustard: 2 tsp.

- 1 Minced garlic clove

- Lemon juice: 1 tsp.

- Honey: half tsp.

- Lemon zest: ¼ tsp.

- Red pepper flakes: ¼ tsp.

- Fresh rosemary: 1 tsp., chopped

- Panko breadcrumbs: 3 tbsp.

- Kosher salt: half tsp.

- Olive oil: 1 tsp.

- 1 skinless salmon fillet (1 pound)

- Chopped walnuts: 3 tbsp.

Instructions

- Let the oven preheat to 425 F.

- In a bowl, add walnuts, oil and panko. In another bowl, add the rest of the ingredients except for fish.

- On a parchment-lined baking tray, place fish and spread the Dijon mixture over fish and add panko mixture on top. Pat to adhere and spray with oil.

- Bake for 8-12 minutes.

- Serve with parsley and lemon.

Mediterranean Meatless & Vegetarian Recipes

Pumpkin Lasagna

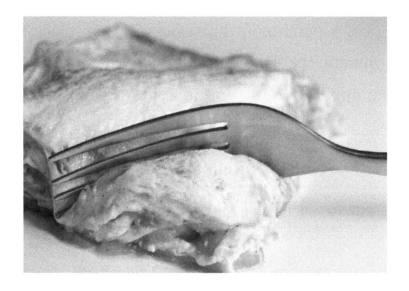

(Prep time: 25 minutes | Cook time: 55 minutes |Servings: 6)

Nutrition: 310 Cal | 12 g Fat |32 g Carbs | 17 g Protein

Ingredients

- 1 Onion, diced

- Olive oil: 2 tsp.

- Sliced mushrooms: half pound

- 1 can of (15 oz.) Pumpkin, solid-pack

- Cream & milk: half cup

- Pepper, to taste

- Cook lasagna noodles: 9 no.

- Shredded parmesan cheese: 3/4 cup

- Salt: half tsp.

- Low-fat ricotta cheese: 1 cup

- Dried sage leaves: 1 tsp.

- Shredded mozzarella cheese: 1 cup

Instructions

- In a skillet, add oil, saute onion, mushrooms with salt until tender.

- In a bowl, add pumpkin, pepper, cream, salt, and sage.

- Take a baking dish, and oil sprays the dish. Spread a half cup of pumpkin mixture on the bottom.

- Add three noodles, add half a cup of pumpkin sauce, and spread.

- Add half of the mushrooms, half a cup of each (mozzarella & ricotta), parmesan cheese (1/4 cup). Repeat the layers, add noodles on top, and sauce.

- Bake for 45 minutes at 375, covered. Uncover it and add the rest of the cheese, bake for 10 to 15 minutes. Let it rest for ten minutes before serving.

Pumpkin Roll-Ups

(Prep time: 20 minutes | Cook time: 45 minutes |Servings: 6)

Nutrition: 313 Cal | 14 g Fat |35 g Carbs | 19 g Protein

Ingredients

The Filling

- Vegan ricotta: 8 oz.

- Garlic powder: half tsp.

- Pumpkin puree: 4 oz.

- Pepper: half tsp.

- Fresh basil: 4 tbsp., chopped

- Salt: half tsp.

The Sauce

- 2 diced cloves of garlic

- Non-dairy milk: 12 oz.

- Vegan butter: 2 tbsp.

- 1 Shallot, chopped

- 3 Sage fresh leaves

- Vegan cream cheese: 2 tbsp.

- Fresh rosemary: 1 sprig, diced

- Vegan broth: 8 oz.

- Flour: 2 tbsp.

The Lasagna

- 10 lasagna noodles

Instructions

- Boil the lasagna noodles until al dente. Drain and rinse with cold water.

- In a bowl, add all ingredients of fillings, mix and set it aside.

- In a pan, saute herbs, garlic, shallots in butter with salt and pepper.

- Cook for 2 to 3 minutes, add milk, flour, and broth, whisk until it boils.

- Turn the heat low and add cream cheese, whisk until it thickens.

- Add lemon juice if you want. Adjust seasonings and turn the heat off.

- Let the oven preheat to 425 F.

- In a casserole dish, add one cup of sauce, add filling (2 tbsp.) on each lasagna noodle, spread it. Roll it and place it in the casserole dish.

- Add the rest of the sauce over noodles. Bake in the oven for 25 minutes.

- Switch on the broil, cook for 2-3 minutes.

- Take it out and rest for five minutes. Serve right away.

Oven-Baked Vegetarian Tacos

(Prep time: 10 minutes | Cook time: 10 minutes |Servings: 4)

Nutrition: 276 Cal | 11 g Fat |13 g Carbs | 12 g Protein

Ingredients

- Chipotle taco lentil meat

- Half sweet onion, diced

- Vegan queso

- Taco shells: 8 crunchy

- Salt, to taste

- Shredded lettuce, as needed

- Cilantro: 4 tbsp., diced

- 1 Lime's juice

Instructions

- Make the lentil taco meat (recipe no. 29), and set it aside.

- Let the oven preheat to 400 F.

- In each taco, add lentil meat and put it in a casserole dish. Add vegan queso to every taco.

- Bake for 7 to 10 minutes.

- In a bowl, toss the cilantro, onion with salt, and lime juice.

- On hot tacos, add lettuce and vegetable mixture. Serve right away.

Chipotle Lentil Taco Meat

(Prep time: 5 minutes | Cook time: 10 minutes |Servings: 6)

Nutrition: 271 Cal | 8 g Fat |11 g Carbs | 12 g Protein

Ingredients

- 1/4 red onion, chopped

- Chipotle peppers: 1 to 2 in adobo, chopped

- Broth: 1/4 cup

- Olive oil: 1 tbsp.

- Adobo sauce: 1 to 2 tbsp., from can

- Taco seasoning: 1 to 2 tbsp.

- Salt & pepper, to taste

- Cooked lentils: 2 ½ cups

Instructions

- In a pan, add oil over medium flame. Saute onion for 2 minutes.

- Add adobe sauce and peppers and cook for 2 minutes.

- Add broth, taco seasonings, and lentils. Cook on low for five minutes.

- Add salt and pepper to taste.

- Serve in tacos.

Mediterranean Pork, Lamb & Beef Recipes

Mediterranean Grilled Pork Roast

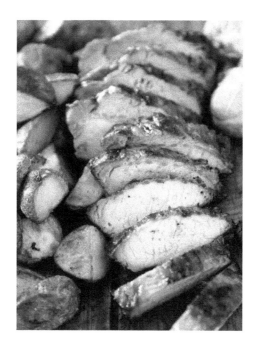

(Prep time: 10 minutes | Cook time: 9 to 10 hours|Servings: 6)

Nutrition: 256 Cal | 9 g Fat |11 g Carbs |24 g Protein

Ingredients

- Fresh sage leaves: 1/4 cup

- Pork loin roast: 4 pounds, boneless

- Salt: 1 tbsp.

- 5 cloves of garlic

- Fresh rosemary leaves: 1/3 cup

- 2 lemons

- Coarse black pepper: 1/4 cup

Instructions

- In a food processor, add all ingredients except for pork. Pulse until fine.

- Coat the pork in the mixture and put it on an indirect heat grill (medium heat).

- Grill, covered for 1-1 ¼, until the internal temperature of the meat reaches 145 F.

- Take off the grill, rest for ten minutes. Serve.

Mediterranean Steak Bites

(Prep time: 40 minutes | Cook time: 10 minutes|Servings: 6)

Nutrition: 370 Cal | 20 g Fat |4 g Carbs |42 g Protein

Ingredients

- Steak: 1.5 lb., cut into half" pieces

- Fresh thyme: half tbsp.

- Fresh rosemary: 1 tsp.

- Grape tomatoes: 1 cup, halved

- Olive oil: 2 to 3 tbsp.

- Dried oregano: half tsp.

- 2 minced garlic cloves

- Cracked pepper: half tsp.

- Lemon juice: 2 tsp.

- Sea salt: half tsp.

- Feta cheese: ⅓ cup

Instructions

- In a ziplock bag, add all ingredients, shake well to coat the steak pieces.

- Keep in the fridge for half an hour.

- In a skillet, add oil on medium flame. Cook steak pieces 2 to 3 minutes on each side.

- Add feta on top and serve with tzatziki sauce.

Mediterranean Beef Casserole

(Prep time: 25 minutes | Cook time: 2 hours|Servings: 6)

Nutrition: 365 Cal | 11 g Fat | 6 g Carbs |23 g Protein

Ingredients

- Stewing steak: 1 lb., cut into large pieces

- Olive oil: 2tbsp.

- 2 red peppers, sliced into large pieces

- 1 Yellow pepper, sliced into large pieces

- Plum tomatoes: 3 cups, quartered

- 2 Heads of garlic, cut in half

- 2 Red onions, sliced into thick wedges

- Sundried tomato paste: 2tbsp.

- Mixed olives: 1 cup, drained

- Red wine: one cup

- Fresh oregano: 6 tbsp.

Instructions

- Let the oven preheat to 375 F.

- In a roasting tin, heat the oil. Sear the meat for five minutes on medium flame and take out on a plate.

- Sauté the peppers and onions for five minutes.

- Add the rest of the ingredients, water (half cup), and beef back in. Bake in the oven for 60 minutes, covered with foil.

- Take off the foil, bake for 60 more minutes. Serve.

Mediterranean Beef with Artichokes

(Prep time: 20 minutes | Cook time: 8 hours|Servings: 6)

Nutrition: 326 Cal | 12 g Fat | 14 g Carbs |24 g Protein

Ingredients

- Grapeseed oil: 1 tbsp.

- 1 Onion, chopped

- Stewing beef: 2 pounds

- 4 minced garlic cloves

- 1 can of (32 oz.) Beef broth

- Dried oregano: 1 tsp.

- 1 can of (15 oz.) Tomato sauce

- Ground cumin: half tsp.

- 1 can of (~15 oz.) Diced tomatoes

- Kalamata olives: half cup, chopped

- Dried parsley: 1 tsp.

- 1 can of (14 oz.) Artichoke hearts, drained & cut in half

- Dried basil: 1 tsp.

- 1 bay leaf

Instructions

- In a pot, add oil over medium flame. Cook beef for 2 minutes on each side.

- In a slow cooker, add the beef with the rest of the ingredients.

- Cook for 7 hours on low, till beef, is tender.

Mediterranean Soup, Pasta & Salad Recipes

Greek Pasta Bake

(Prep time: 20 minutes | Cook time: 25 minutes |Servings: 8)

Nutrition: 398 Cal | 10 g Fat | 47 g Carbs |34 g Protein

Ingredients

- Whole grain penne pasta: 3-1/3 cups, uncooked

- 1 Can of (~15 oz.) Drained diced tomatoes

- Dried basil: 1 tsp.

- 1 pack of (10 oz.) Chopped spinach

- Chicken breast: 4 cups, cubed & cooked

- 1 Can of (~15 oz. Each) drained sliced olives

- Crumbled feta cheese: half cup

- Red onion: 1/4 cup, thinly sliced

- 1 can of (29 oz.) Tomato sauce

- Chopped green pepper: 1/4 cup

- Dried oregano: 1 tsp.

- Shredded mozzarella cheese: 1 cup

Instructions

- Cook pasta as per package instructions.

- Take out in a bowl, and add all vegetables.

- Toss and put in an oil sprayed (13 by 9") baking dish

- Add cheese on top.

- Bake at 400 F until cheese melts. Serve with fresh herbs on top.

Farmers Market Pasta

(Prep time: 20 minutes | Cook time: 20 minutes |Servings: 6)

Nutrition: 338 Cal | 9 g Fat | 46 g Carbs |23 g Protein

Ingredients

- Whole wheat linguine: 9 oz., uncooked

- 2 carrots, sliced thin

- 2 zucchinis, sliced thin

- Fresh mushrooms: half-pound, sliced

- 1 Red onion, diced

- 2 Minced garlic cloves

- Fresh asparagus: 1 pound, 2-inch pieces

- Cooked ham: 2 cups, cubed

- Cream: 1 cup

- Fresh basil: 2 tbsp.

- Chicken broth: 2/3 cup

- Grated parmesan cheese: half cup

- Petite peas: 1 cup

- Pepper: 1/4 tsp.

Instructions

- Cook pasta as per package instructions.

- In a pan, add oil to coat the pan. Saute onion for three minutes.

- Add garlic, squash and mushrooms for 4 to 5 minutes.

- Add broth and cream, let it boil and deglaze the pan. Turn the heat low and cook for five minutes.

- Add pepper, peas, basil and ham. Heat it through.

- Add this mixture to pasta, add cheese. Mix well and serve.

Couscous Salad

(Prep time: 15 minutes | Cook time: 15 minutes |Servings: 8)

Nutrition: 315 Cal | 9 g Fat | 32 g Carbs |23 g Protein

Ingredients

- Pearl couscous: 1 1/3 cups

- Olive oil: 1 tbsp.

- Cherry tomatoes: 10 oz. Halved

- 2 minced garlic cloves

- Sun-dried tomatoes (in oil): 4 oz., chopped

- Juice from half lemon

- 1 Can of (14-oz.) Chickpeas, rinsed

- Pesto: ¼ to 1/2 cup

- Salt & black pepper, to taste

- 5 basil leaves, chopped

- Red pepper flakes, to taste

- Arugula: 1 cup

Instructions

- In a pan, add oil and saute garlic with couscous. Stir until browned, add water and cook with a lid.

- Take off the lid and fluff with a fork. Add pesto, all tomatoes and mix for 3 to 5 minutes on low.

- Add the rest of the ingredients except for the greens. Toss well.

- Add basil, arugula, and toss.

- Serve right away or serve chilled.

Hummus & Greek Salad

(Prep time: 10 minutes | Cook time: 0 minutes |Servings: 1)

Nutrition: 422 Cal | 29 g Fat | 30 g Carbs |10 g Protein

Ingredients

- Arugula: 2 cups

- Sliced cucumber: ⅓ cup

- Hummus: ¼ cup

- Red onion: 1 tbsp., chopped

- Cherry tomatoes: ⅓ cup, halved

- Olive oil: 1 ½ tbsp.

- 1 Whole-wheat pita (4-inch)

- Red-wine vinegar: 2 tsp.

- Feta cheese: 1 tbsp.

- Ground pepper, to taste

Instructions

- In a bowl, add all ingredients except for pita and hummus.

- Toss well and serve with pita & hummus.

Mediterranean Dessert Recipes

Blueberry Muffins

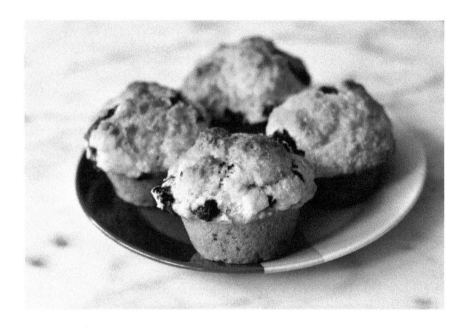

(Prep time: 10 minutes | Cook time: 18 minutes |Servings: 24)

Nutrition: 176 Cal |8 g Fat |13 g Carbs |6 g Protein

Ingredients

Dry ingredients

- Salt: 1 tsp.

- All-purpose flour: 2 cups

- Baking powder: 6 tsp.

- Blueberries: 2 cups

- Whole wheat flour: 2 cups

- Sugar: 2/3 cup

Wet ingredients

- Milk: 2 cups

- 2 eggs

- Olive oil: 2/3 cup

Instructions

- Let the oven preheat to 400 F.

- In a bowl, add all dry ingredients, mix and add blueberries.

- In another bowl, add wet ingredients, add wet to dry ingredients.

- Mix to combine, do not over mix.

- Pour into oil spray muffin tin, bake for 18 minutes.

Chocolate Avocado Pudding

(Prep time: 5 minutes | Cook time: 0 minutes |Servings: 4)

Nutrition: 324Cal | 23 g Fat |34 g Carbs |6 g Protein

Ingredients

- Cacao powder: 1/3 cup

- 2 chilled avocado

- Vanilla extract: 2 tsp.

- Coconut milk: half cup

- Maple syrup: 1/3 cup

Instructions

- Cut the avocados in half and take out the pit.

- In a food processor, add avocado flesh with other ingredients.

- Pulse on high until smooth. Adjust sweetness.

- Pour the pudding into serving bowls and serve right away.

Greek Honey Cake with Pistachios

(Prep time: 10 minutes | Cook time: 30 minutes |Servings: 6)

Nutrition: 379 Cal | 10 g Fat |67 g Carbs |8 g Protein

Ingredients

- Low-fat Greek yogurt: 1 cup

- 1 Orange's zest

- Ground almonds: 5 tbsp.

- 5 eggs

- Coarse semolina: 1 cup

- 1 lemon's zest

- Granulated sugar: 2 cups

- Baking powder: 2 tsp.

- Olive oil: ¾ cup + 1 tbsp.

- All-purpose flour: 1 ¼ cup

For Honey Pistachio Syrup

- 1 lemon's juice

- salted pistachios (shelled): 1 1/4 cup

- 2 oranges' juice

- Runny honey: 1 ¼ cup

Instructions

- Let the oven preheat to 350 F.

- Oil spray a 9 by 13 pan and dust with flour.

- In a bowl, add all batter ingredients except for almonds. Mix to combine.

- Pour the batter into the pan.

- Bake for 25-30 minutes until inserted toothpick comes out clean.

- Take out and let it cool.

- In a pan, toast the pistachios on medium flame. Once fragrant, add honey.

- Add lemon juice and orange juice. Boil for 1-2 minutes.

- Pierce the cake with a fork all over and pour the syrup over the cake.

- Sprinkle almonds on top.

- Serve.

Mediterranean Dips, Spreads, Sauces & Snacks Recipes

Roasted Chickpeas

(Prep time: 5 minutes | Cook time: 30 minutes |Servings: 2)

Nutrition: 498 Cal | 28 g Fat |43.7 g Carbs |15.8 g Protein

Ingredients

- Lemon juice: 2 tsp.

- 2 cans of (15 oz.) Chickpeas, rinsed

- Garlic powder: half tsp.

- Red wine vinegar: 2 tsp.

- Kosher salt: 1 tsp.

- Olive oil: 2 tbsp.

- Dried oregano: 1 tsp.

- Cracked black pepper: half tsp.

Instructions

- Let the oven preheat to 425 F.

- On a parchment lined baking tray, spread the chickpeas.

- Roast for ten minutes, stir and roast for ten more minutes.

- In a bowl, add the rest of the ingredients and whisk. Add hot chickpeas in the sauce toss to coat.

- Spread on a baking tray and roast for ten minutes.

- Serve cooled or warm.

Quinoa Granola

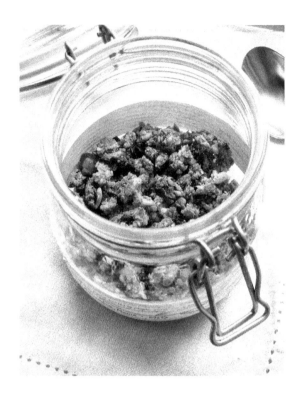

(Prep time: 5 minutes | Cook time: 25 minutes |Servings: 7)

Nutrition: 332 Cal | 6.3 g Fat |30 g Carbs |9 g Protein

Ingredients

- Rolled oats (old-fashioned): 1 cup,

- Sea salt, a pinch

- White quinoa: half cup

- Coconut oil: 3 1/2 tbsp.

- Raw almonds: 2 cups, chopped

- Maple syrup: 1/4 cup

- Coconut sugar: 1 tbsp.

Instructions

- Let the oven preheat to 340 F.

- In a bowl, add all ingredients except for coconut oil and maple syrup. Stir well.

- In a pan, add maple syrup and oil. Heat for 2-3 minutes and whisk to combine.

- Pour this mixture over dry ingredients, and coat well.

- Spread on a baking tray in one even layer.

- Bake for 20 minutes, take out, and stir.

- Bake again for 5 to 10 minutes; make sure not to burn.

- Serve.

Spinach Walnut Greek Yogurt Dip

(Prep time: 10 minutes | Cook time: 0 minutes |Servings: 8)

Nutrition: 52 Cal | 3.7 g Fat |1.9 g Carbs |3.5 g Protein

Ingredients

- Baby spinach: 2 cups

- Chopped parsley: half cup

- Kosher salt, to taste

- Walnuts: ¾ cup, finely chopped

- Black pepper, as needed

- 1-2 minced garlic cloves

- Greek yogurt: 2 cups

- Lemon juice: 1 tbsp.

- Dry mint: 1 tsp.

- Olive oil: 2 tbsp.

Instructions

- In a pot, boil water. In a bowl, add ice water.

- Add spinach in boiling water for ten seconds, and then place in ice water. Take out on paper towels.

- In a bowl, add the rest of the ingredients with blanched spinach.

- Season with salt and pepper.

Beet Hummus

(Prep time: 15 minutes | Cook time: 0 minutes |Servings: 8)

Nutrition: 224 Cal | 14 g Fat |20 g Carbs |7 g Protein

Ingredients

- Tahini: 3 tbsp.

- Canned chickpeas: 4 cups, rinsed

- Olive oil: ⅓ cup

- 1 Minced garlic clove

- 1 beet: cooked, & chopped

- Lemon juice: ¼ cup

- Salt & black pepper, to taste

Instructions

- In a food processor, add all ingredients. Pulse until smooth, adjust seasoning.

- Serve right away for a drizzle of olive oil on top.

Conclusion

Congratulations on finishing this book.

If you really want to improve your lifestyle, the Mediterranean diet is the best diet for you. In addition to being one of the healthiest and most balanced, it is also one of the largest in the choice of raw materials. At the base of a self-respecting Mediterranean diet there is a considerable consumption of fruit and vegetables, an intake of a lot of water and the reduction of red meat in our diet. It is very important to learn how to follow these little tips if you want to get great results from the first weeks. I hope you were satisfied with my recipes.

Enjoy.

Lightning Source UK Ltd.
Milton Keynes UK
UKHW020750030621
384855UK00001B/42